Behind The Mask

Hannah Dee

I hate it when something relatively insignificant consumes your every thought.

Over & over in my mind I keep thinking about it, but nothing I say to myself makes any difference. It's over & done with, a blimp in time really; but it's on my mind constantly.

Apologies have been made & explanations given but I still feel bad. Guilty even ... but for what?

Copyright © 2012 Hannah Dee

All rights reserved.

ISBN: 9781723791987

DEDICATION

FOR MY LITTLE LOVES.
YOU HELP ME TO LOVE, LEARN AND GROW.
MY WORLD IS RICHER FOR HAVING MET YOU.

AND TO MY DEAR FRIEND BELINDA WHO I MISS EVERY DAY
XXXX

I AM

I am emotional, hyper, moody and easily destroyed by words spoken in a moment of madness.

I am lost in a sea of faces, yet stand out in a crowd like a neon light.

I can lose my voice when I've not spoken for days, yet find my strength in helping others find theirs.

I am a contradiction.

I am insensitive.

I am compassionate.

I am humble.

I am brave.

I am everything you told me I could not be and I am accepting of it all.

Embracing wisdom and embracing the flaws of life.

Chasing dreams that will break me.

Chasing life as it passes me by.

Living rather than existing.

I am.

I am.

I am.

Behind The Mask

EARLY DAYS....

My life began on February 19th, 1979, in Tasmania. I was the first-born daughter for my parents and their second child.

My parents were married for 23 years. My mother and father were married in 1976 just after my brother was born; she was 18 at the time and my father was 24. My little sister arrived in 1981 and in July 1987 my younger brother was born.

For as long I can remember my mother has suffered from back problems. When she was 16 she fell off a ladder at work. My father was a self-employed wood merchant and hay bale hauler. I rarely saw him most days as he was up at dawn and home after dark. He was a big drinker.

I don't remember having a happy childhood. Although I come from a large family, I always felt alone and afraid. I always felt like the odd one out; the black sheep of the family. I was depressed by the time I was in grade 6. I had no friends and was always bullied and picked on by my peers; If my teachers contacted my mother with their concerns; she would always tell them I was making up stories or saying things for attention.

I always wished that I would get kidnapped or taken away because she treated me like a slave, abused me emotionally and physically and made me feel like I had wronged her by being born.

My father could see how badly my mother treated me but was powerless to stop it.

By the age of 14 I was the local babysitter. It was my escape from the family home. I got close to one of the mums I babysat for. I used to look after her 2 children on a regular basis and when she saw me struggling with life, she would take me away for the weekend telling my mother that I was helping her look after her kids. My mother hated this and tried to sever the relationship.

Eventually she succeeded and I was replaced as babysitter by another young girl that needed saving.

Home life was never much fun for me. I was the cook, the cleaner, the laundry attendant, the live in babysitter for my little brother Nicholas. My mother never let me join any after school activities, or have friends stay over. She controlled everything about my life. I never went to college, barely finished year 10.

My PCOS (poly cystic ovarian syndrome) caused me a lot of trouble and I spent most of that year in and out of hospital. I had a burst appendix that same year that sent my stomach septic and I needed 3 months off school to recuperate. My mother never finished year 8 so she didn't encourage or support me to continue my studies.

When I was 16 I got my first job as a retail assistant. I loved my job! It gave me freedom to be me and I had my own money and could have friends of my own.

My first relationship was with an older man, and after 6 months together I got pregnant with my first son.

I was only 17 at the time, but had turned 18 by the time he was born. During the pregnancy my mother told me repeatedly that I was going to fail and be a bad mother. She drove me to the family planning clinic many times, during the first trimester, and told me to get rid of it. (meaning the baby) but I wouldn't do it.

Refusing to have my baby terminated only infuriated her more and life became progressively worse for me.

I moved out of home when my baby was 3 months old but I struggled to keep my finances in order and had to rely on my parents to bail me out of debt.

I had never been taught how to save or budget my money. And most of what I earned from my job in retail had gone to her as board and food. Because she bailed me out of debt so many times my mother was at my home most days.

The bond between my son and myself was damaged due to her constant criticism and interference. When I was diagnosed with post-natal depression in 1998 she told me it was because I had made a mistake in having him. She always reminded me of my mistakes in life, and the debt that I owed her financially. She was controlling my life to the point that I couldn't survive without her by my side. It affected me mentally and emotionally and I was suffering from major depression. I felt I had not option other than to leave Tasmania and try to start my life over again.

In February 2003 I made the decision to leave Tasmania.

I moved to Melbourne and moved in with my older brother. My mother refused to let me leave with my son. After some negotiation I left him behind with the belief that once I had settled with my brother I would return to collect him. But in my short absence she applied to the family court for full custody; stating that I had abandoned him.

The court process lasted 8 months before I was awarded custody again and he came to live with me in Melbourne. By then he was almost 7 years old.

Once I had my own home, life was finally starting to become easier and happier for both of us.

In January 2004 I met and married my second sons father. We divorced in 2006, This impacted greatly on my mental health and I needed a lot of in hospital support to help with depression and later a diagnosis of BPD (borderline personality disorder).

I was intent on ending my life at that time and was unable to see any good coming from my life. In March 2008 my now ex-husband passed away from complications resulting from surgery.

This destroyed me; I had major guilt and felt like I had failed him as a wife. I felt that I didn't deserve life after being such a horrible human being. I didn't deserve happiness, I didn't deserve, peace, I didn't deserve any kind of goodness in my life – including my children.

I made the heartbreaking decision to place my children in voluntary foster care so that I could seek support and recovery for my mental illness, depression, anxiety and suicidal ideation.

I had no control over my actions at this time and after an almost successful suicide attempt my beautiful boys were placed in foster care together by order of the court.

When my mother found out that my boys were being looked after by a stranger, she applied to have my eldest placed back into her care. She was given the opportunity to also take my youngest but she didn't want to. So he sadly went to a new carer by himself and had supervised contact with me 3 times a week.

I struggled greatly with my mental health off and on for the next 4 years off and on. During this time however, I never stopped fighting for my boys to return home.

Although I knew they were being well cared for and looked after, I still needed to have them return home to me so that I could continue on my road to recovery. Without them to wake up for, I was struggling to find a purpose in life.

After some time of stability in my mental state my youngest finally came back home to me. In total he had been in care for a little over 11 months; thankfully the majority of that time was spent with the same carers.

Whilst in hospital recovering from my many crises I started writing down how I felt. It was the only way I could find a voice for what I was feeling that didn't make me sound like I was attention seeking. It started a whole new chapter (metaphorically) in my life. Chronicling my life in poem was helping me heal and learn my triggers.

Once I started noticing a pattern in my behavior and saw what was and wasn't helping me I was able to advocate for myself and I took back the control that mental illness had taken from me for so many years.

Others started reading what I had written and told me that it had helped them to seek treatment and they had taken a particular poem to their doctor and from reading it; they were able to form a plan to get supports in place.

For the first time in my life I was hearing good things about myself. It took a long time for me to realize that they actually meant it; they weren't just saying these things to make me feel better. Slowly life started to change and look hopeful for the first time.

 All the abuse I had suffered was starting to count for something, so I used it to educate others about the importance of NOT keeping silent when something or someone is hurting you. Turning my pain into a lesson helped me move on and grow as a person.

In 2012 I published my first book titled *'Death Didn't Want Me ... Now I Have Life'* Since then I have published another two books.

My second book was written while pregnant with my youngest son and is titled *'Cracks In My Reflection'* and my latest book; released in March 2016 is simply titled *'Taken'* and is full of content that is related to the impacts of my babies being taken away. It gives the perspective of how heartbreaking it is to say goodbye to your babies when they are screaming at you that they want to stay.

Although I now understand why they were taken from me, the scars left behind have contributed to who I am today. A strong, determined fighter that uses her experiences to educate others on mental health and forgiveness.

I am a public speaker and speak at forums, functions, events about what I have learnt from falling so low. I am a member on numerous consumer committees that help mental health carers/consumers/nominated persons gain access to clear informative information about their treatment options and legal rights.

All my boys have learnt from me that no matter what life throws at them – I am always and WILL ALWAYS be there to help them back up again. I let them know that it's okay to make mistakes as long as you learn from them.

We all keep a jar close by that is full of the positive things in life that we tend to forget when the world is crumbling around us. We sit and read them together and pretty soon; we all have smiles on our faces remembering.

I don't hide my struggles with mental health from them – and they are so much more caring, considerate and empathetic towards others because of it. I'm proud of all three of them and hope to give my learned life experience of trauma and heartache to other children that might not be as lucky as my boys are.

I know that Lily, my first foster care child, is thriving from being with us; and although she may not be my child by blood – in my eyes she is my daughter and I will do anything and everything to help her get from life what she deserves.

As a mother, I cannot comprehend how or why my own mother treated me the way she did. This is what drives me to be the mother I am today and what pushes me to go outside my comfort zone and be someone to a child that has no one.

I never want to make you feel alone.
I never want to make cry.
I never want to see tears coming from your eyes.
I never thought it would be you telling me these lies.

Will you let me leave without trying to get me to stay?
Are you just gonna let us die right here?
Nothing left but pain & fears?
Will we really be apart?
Leaving bruises on my heart?

We always fought because it meant so much.
Arguments turned into silence and days of nothing but frosted glares.
Too stubborn to back down.
Too proud to say I'm sorry first.

Will you let me leave without trying to get me to stay?
Are you just gonna let us die right here?
Nothing left but pain & fears?
Will we really be apart?
Leaving bruises on my heart?

MOTHER

Today is April 20th, 2018. It was a year ago today that I last had any contact with my mother.

Our last conversation was via text and I told her 'Hope life treats you well. I'm done'.

She has made no attempt to call me or try and undo what was done.

As a mother myself; I cannot understand nor comprehend how she so easily turned her back on me. I would NEVER let my child go, no matter what.

You're meant to argue with your parents, be upset, disappointed, and even angry with them at some point. But they are meant to be in your face and telling you that no matter what. you are their child and they will never let you go.

They are meant to hold you when you fall and celebrate when you win and dry your tears when you fall apart and cry.

She just turned her back and pretended like she never had 2 daughters. Only 1.

When my sons are trying to push me away I just push them back harder and keep telling them that nothing they do or say will ever make me walk away and wipe my hands of their existence. But that's the difference between her and me I guess; I'm proud of my children and don't regret having them. My life is richer because of them. I bet that she can't say that.

And in case your curious what her last words to me were, I will tell you.

Her text said *'I have enough shit going on without this too & I have people here & can't talk. Message me whatever excuse you have because right now I've got nothing to say to you!'*

The 'shit' she was talking about was me winning an award that celebrated me as a mother and the obstacles I had overcome in life to achieve the recognition.

If this was my child ... I'd scream about it from the rooftops for all to hear & boring people with the details! I would be THAT Mum; the one always boasting about her kids but I'd be okay with that because my child's success is a reflection of me. I see nothing wrong with that.

Now; Let me make something clear. I don't miss her. I don't want to reconcile and I don't want a relationship with her again. Life is easier without her and I strive to be the opposite of everything she ever was and did to me for my own kids.

But a whole year

huh? I can't imagine not being in my child's life for that long. What a failure I'd be as a mother.

Everyone told me I was way too young,
Go out & live your life,
Go & have some fun.
But fun isn't what I was looking for,
I needed someone to love
That was mine for sure.

Now I've got three beautiful boys
The son's in my day.
My reason for breathing,
My purpose.
My life.

ME AND THE UNIVERSE

I did a talk in 2017 at a public forum about my healing journey (despise the word recovery) and I remember seeing a young girl come in about 3 mins or so after I'd started speaking; but she stayed till the end and came up to me afterwards and asked if she could give me a hug. We hugged and she said 'thank you' and walked away.

I tried to find her before I left the forum but couldn't. There was something about her hug that made me want to reach inside her heart and take away her pain. Everyone I asked didn't recognize her or hadn't even noticed she was there.

Something about the girl was nagging me all night, couldn't stop thinking about her.

Late the next night I got a message from her.

She told me that she had been on her way home after a bad session with her case manager and didn't know what made her walk in to the room but she wanted to tell me something.

She told me "I had decided I was going home to kill myself; but now I want to get better so I can help people like you do".

We've stayed in touch and she's doing good.

And I'm so happy I dragged my arse along to the forum that day; because I'd wanted to stay home and let the haters win.

The universe works in mysterious ways.

YESTERDAY AND TODAY

Yesterday I cried a little, then I cried some more. The day before that I cried a lot and lots more the day before that. Sometimes I feel like I'm 'normal' whatever that means; then some days I feel like the world is closing in on me and that means it's making everything seem so small.

Today I laughed with my friends and we made plans to meet again next week; I answered the phone and managed some calls; but I couldn't do it yesterday.

Sometimes I get this overwhelming urge to hurt myself so that I can be the one in control, but I keep myself busy and hope that it passes. Not giving in to the urges sometimes gives me guilt and makes it worse than it was before but it's part of who I am inside. Still searching, still hurting, still wanting, still needing. But mostly it's like I'm wounded from war but no one can see my scars, and I feel I've got to rip myself open to find the beginning and the end.

Today I made it without doing that and I hope tomorrow I can do it too, but depression and suicidal ideation doesn't come with a warning, just a sudden and an intense feeling and emotion.

But I can mark another day off the calendar that I have made it through and now the number stands at 3,204.

Every day I feel these things but I don't want to die, it's just a part inside that makes me, some days I can laugh and other days I cry.

Mental illness is nothing to be ashamed of. It's just a part of who I am. Tomorrow I will probably cry a little or maybe even a lot, but I'm not worried and neither should you be, because I always remember to remember that 'you got this Hannah! Fight on you friggen rockstar' and I say 'thank you! Damn it! I will!'

IT'S NOT OKAY

Spreading hate is *NOT OKAY*.

Sharing photos/images that are not your property is *NOT OKAY*.

Deliberately spreading abusive messages is *NOT OKAY*.

Naming and shaming someone because you disagree with their opinion, thoughts, statement or behavior IS *NOT OKAY*.

Posting slanderous statements about someone else IS *NOT OKAY*.

Sadly, we live in a world that enables us to screen shot everything that goes out on the internet and even what should be personal/private property is captured and used against another in ways that are inappropriate and can have devastating consequences.

Do you know how many people a day commit suicide in Australia alone as a direct result of cyber bullying?...3

That is 3 too many. The national average of suicides a day in Australia is 8.

8 people a day take their own lives and that breaks my heart. When is enough, enough?

I have personally been affected by cyber bullying this last week and as someone who suffers from mental illness, let me tell you, it's damn hard to ignore it.

It has pushed me to my limits and left me sobbing hysterically for hours at a time when I see the hate and the ignorance of the people spreading it.

Lives are being destroyed every day because all it takes is for one person to start and then someone else starts and then you see others start to follow. It grows; it gets so out of control that now I start having a panic attack every time my phone makes a noise.

But as hard as it might be I refuse to let them win!

They can say what they like and spread their vile abuse all over social media! I am an adult; old enough to realize that the people behind this are trolls with nothing better to do. Doesn't mean that is still doesn't hurt and open up old wounds.

But I worry about my children; especially my 11-year-old. And although he doesn't have a mobile phone or any social media accounts. He only has to google my name and it's all there. His peers have these accounts and they show him what people are saying, and most of the time it is all innocent when they ask him 'why did they say that about your mum?' or 'look at this!' but it is not innocent when my son reads it. It affects him just as much as it affects me, only he doesn't want me to see it so he hides it.

But he's suffering and I can see it. What can I do as a parent to help him get rid the 'shame' that he now feels because someone showed him this hatred about his mum that he can't see? What can I do as an adult to help him understand that sadly, this is considered normal nowadays?

So last night I sat him down and I tried explaining to him that not everyone has the same heart that he does and that people thrive on this sort of drama. I told him that even though it isn't true what they are saying, other people will believe it and there is nothing we can do about it.

What makes me angry, what really hurts the most, is when he turned around and said to me 'I'm sorry I nominated you mum of the year and you won because you don't deserve all this hate'. How devastated am I to hear him say that? How devastated is he to be thinking that?

This is not okay! He feels like he is to blame for this bullying because he wanted everyone to know how amazing he thinks I am and I am completely heartbroken.

Knowing that 99% of the bullying has come from my 'family' hurts him even more because he can't understand how 'family' can say such horrible, cruel things to each other.

Families are meant to love each other! And yes, in reality family is meant to protect you and love you and spare you from unnecessary pain – but mine won't.

This is where I am different to them. I show my children what a family is and I teach them about respect and about watching out for each other and that it is not acceptable to hurt each other because you can't control how the other person reacts or feels.

We as a family love each other regardless of our flaws, our mistakes, our beliefs or our opinions and as a mother I cannot comprehend how or when it would ever be acceptable to sit back and watch someone spread hate of any form about any of my children.

Sadly, this is obviously not the case when it comes to the woman that gave birth to me, because it is her and her followers that are inflicting this pain on us.

When you become that target of someone's hatred, nothing you do will stop them from trying to cause you as much pain as possible. Whether it starts because of the misuse of a word in a sentence, or the innocent words of an 11-year-old boy spoken out of love for his mum, the bully won't stop until they see you down on the ground and begging for them to stop.

If they see weakness they will only pounce again and this time bring even more people in to the 'game' to try and break you down completely.

I thought that I had faced all of my demons before, and I thought that a truce had been signed off on and sealed, never to be opened again but it looks like I was wrong.

I have never been more ashamed of the blood that runs through my veins that I am today. The DNA that I have sadly passed onto my children, but I will not let them become the monsters that other generations have become! I will show them what love, respect, empathy, integrity, compassion and simple kindness is, and this current vicious cycle of destruction to others will die.

Children need empowerment to create change, build them up so that they can be better than those who have been before them. Teach them that not everyone in this world is capable of hurting others, and lead by example and be the change that you want them to be.

Fighting hate with hate will never have a winner, only casualties of the war. I refuse to be a number that becomes a statistic on a page. Stop for a few minutes and take a look around you and watch what is happening in your own world, and if you see that someone you know is part of this growing epidemic of cyber bullying, sit them down and start a healthy conversation.

Life is hard enough, without all the other complications and there are already too many lost souls because of the cyber bullying.

STOP THE HATE...

This might not change anything, but I have to do something to try and stop the hate.

I'm not perfect. I've never claimed to be. I've made mistakes, had some pretty shitty things happen to me and I've probably not been the best I can be at times. But throughout everything that life has given me; there has always been one thing that I AM good at and that is being a mum!

Finding out that some people feel the need to try and bring me down for being acknowledged as a good mum is just sad.

People can change. People can learn from their mistakes, they can go on and do great things. They can even be better people.

The past is the past and nothing can change it, the future is what matters and the influences you choose to make in it make you who you are. So maybe instead of living in the past, people should start living in the moment, here and now and lift each other up instead of trying to tear others down.

Mental illness is not a choice. Actions, reactions and consequences when someone is mentally unwell should never be used as a weapon to inflict further pain.

I for one am tired of all the negativity that is projected out onto others when they get the opportunity to shine.

Stop the hate. There is so much already in this messed up world we live in, why create more?

Why?

Would you stand in front of your loved one with a single bullet in a chamber of 6 and aim it at them every time you told them they weren't good enough?

No you wouldn't.

Every time you bring them down, taunt them, tease them or lecture them about mental health remember this.

You are playing a deadly game of Russian roulette and next time it may just be the chamber that holds the bullet.

Your words are just as powerful as the bullet in that gun.

Choose them wisely.

METAPHOR OF SELF WORTH.

I'm high up on the shelf, above the bargains and the discounts. I've been picked up many times and examined by many prying eyes. I've had my faults pointed out so many times, that I stopped counting at 95.

I've been laughed at, teased, poked at and prodded so violently; that I've even got the bruises to prove it. I'm covered in dust and smothered in fingerprints. I'm in need of a good soaking or two. But every night as the day draws to a close, I crave time alone away from curious faces that are passing by.

I look back up at the highest shelf and wonder if i can make it back up there again. But just as I'm about to give up; when I'm almost at the top, I look behind me and see how far I've come and how little I have to go. Once I'm back where I belong - high up on the shelf; I can relax and be myself once more.

You see ... up here I'm the protector of all the things that surround me. I'm the first to be picked on, picked over or abused; because I'm the biggest thing on this shelf. The easy target.

But every night I make a choice - to stay where I've been left, forgotten by the last hands that touched me or i can pick myself up, dust myself off and climb back up to where I belong.

Up where I can shine when the light hits me just right, I can look menacing when the light isn't quite right, and I can just blend into the background when I want to.

Up here I know my worth - I'm not a bargain nor a discount. I'm top dollar and worth every penny! But down there I'm lost in the confusion and my value is gone from the ticket.

Know your worth.
Know your value.
Know your importance.
Know your place.
Know that the top shelf is where you belong!

Shining on regardless of what others chose to see in me

Hannah Dee

MY HORMONES ARE WHACKY

My Hormones are whacky,
They make me feel tacky.
I'm up & i'm down and I'm spinning around,
I laugh & I cry;
God I wish I knew why!
No more pms;
But I'm sure there's a test
To check if I'm crazy or just really lazy.

My motivation is gone!
Disappeared it is zip.
And my favourite jeans so sad they did rip.
No longer fit over my thunder thighs,
Due to my lack of exercise.
I eat more junk food than I should,
But god they make it
TASTE SO GOOD!

My Hormones are whacky,
They make me feel tacky.
No longer clothes fit Oh god! There's a zit!
I'm hot then I'm cold and angry I'm told,
When I have conversation it's like an invasion.
The prickles they start and I cough when I fart,
My face it turns red
And I wanna hide in my bed!

My Hormones are whacky,
They make me feel tacky.
I'm always so tired But I can never sleep,
Lay sleepless for hours
Sick of those bloody sheep!
My shower starts hot, Then I turn it to cold.
Hot flushes galore,
I CAN'T TAKE ANYMORE

Do you sometimes think that life isn't fair?
Why can't you seem to get anywhere?
You try & try & try & try
But you still feel like you're just waiting to die?

Chorus:
Put your hands up if u got a label
Put your hand up if ya a little unstable
Put your hands up if ur a little cray cray,
Put your hands up if its gonna be the day aye!

Sometimes life don't treat you right
and knocks you down so you've gotta fight.
When you're down, down on the ground
that's when you see who's stickin around.

Chorus:

Livin life with labels
doesn't have to mean you can't be able,
You can be amazing, You can inspiring...
and you don't need no diploma requirin.

Chorus:

Let your lessons become your teacher
even if it means you sound like a preacher.
Get out there and tell your story,
This is your time, your moment of glory!
Believe in your individuality and embrace the person
you're destined to be.

Chorus:

It's not always how it's s'posed to be,
Life is unfair in reality.
But believe that it can be wonderful
Just gotta find your wonderwall.

Put your hands up, Put your hands up,
Put your hands up, Put your hands up

Chorus:

Sometimes life don't treat you right
and knocks you down so you've gotta fight.
When you're down, down on the ground
that's when you see who's stickin around.

LOSING CONTROL

I've been broken before
But one things for sure,
I'm not givin you that power over me no more!

So just keep on leavin.
Keep right on walkin away,
I'm tired of fightin, there's nothin left in me to say.

You didn't love me.
You only wanted me to stay;
So I could take the pain of your loneliness away.

I've made excuses for my tears
I've been creating them for years,
Trying to keep up the lie But in reality I just wanted to die.

 But the hell you put me through
I could never do to you,
Because it's just not there in me To bring someone to their knees.

You dragged me through the mud!
You threw me under the bus,
You ran over me with a ten tonne truck; But still I got back up!

Yes babe I've been broken before,
But one thing is for sure,
I ain't lettin you have that control over me anymore!

THE TAUNTING

Words are the ammunition.
Memories are the torture.
Regret is the abuser.
The taunting of this night.

Hours creep in twisted humour.
Silence not near or far.
Questionings that fight what is.
The taunting of this night.

Weakened body of helplessness.
Mind of madness with no escape.
Wretched knowing once forgotten.
The taunting of this night.

Elapsed recollection of happy.
Disturbing peace of mind.
Failings of the contented me.
The taunting of this night.

SAVING A LIFE

I saved somebody's life tonight.

I talked him out of suicide and into getting the help he needed.

I was terrified of saying the wrong thing, or of letting him know that I was upset.

The entire time I felt like I was holding my breath - almost too scared to gulp the air I needed into my lungs. I heard his speech start to slur and his breathing become heavy; and I kept reminding him to breathe in and out, in and out ...

He kept apologizing for keeping me awake and for making me worry. But I'm glad he did. Because if I'd let my phone go unanswered, he wouldn't be here. He's in the hospital now, where he needs to be. He's stable but not quite out of the woods. The next few days are going to be tough but I'm going to be with him every step of the way.

This was the hardest thing that I have ever done. Never ever EVER underestimate the power your voice has to help another. When the light has gone, and only darkness remains; your voice can help them find their way to safety.

T

What would you do if a child was standing in front of you hysterical and saying 'I can't take it anymore, I'm better off dead'? 'I should commit suicide and do everyone a favour'.

Would you calm them down and try to get them to tell you what's going on? Would you call their parents and get them to come pick them up?

What if YOU are the parent and the child saying those things is YOURS?

The world stops. Everything happens in slow motion and you can't stop the tears that spring to your eyes from falling. You grab hold of your child and hold them tight and tell them everything will be okay. Just breathe in and out for now, just breathe in and out.

All I could think was Give me your pain, give me your hurt; I can take it! I can take anything except that.

Terrified and scared were all I felt.

I can talk others out of suicide; have a never ending list of things to say to someone that's crying out for help. But I had no words to offer him because it's never something I ever thought I'd need to do.

This happened to us yesterday afternoon and the fear that runs through my veins every time he leaves my sight feels like it's crippling me. I can't breathe until he's back in the room and sitting with us in the lounge.

I'm trained for situations like this, but that meant nothing in the moment.

There were no signs that he was struggling, he came home Happy from school every day. He did his homework and never baulked at going out the door to school in the mornings. He's never said anything was wrong and I never saw it coming.

We've been to see the doctor and organised some counselling through the school so hopefully things are under control again for now.

As a Mum, as a mental health worker, and as an advocate for the rights of everyone ... please tell your children that it's okay to not be okay. Talk to them, love them and most importantly do not judge them! Thankfully he is going to be okay and nothing too serious came from this sudden, frightening breakdown that he had. But had I not been here when he got home? ... I shudder at the thought.

Pay attention to what they do say and what they don't. Let them know that no matter what they have to say, it's important and it matters. Hug them tight and remind them they mean the world to you so that they will remember when their world becomes dark.

2017

In April of this year (2017) two things happened that changed the direction of my life.

The first thing was our little foster baby went back home. She had been with us for 46 weeks and 4 days. She had her first Christmas with us, we celebrated her first birthday together and we got to witness her crawling for the first time.

But the pain my heart felt when she left is like nothing I've ever felt before. All of us felt the loss for a long time after she had gone. We were promised visits and the chance to let go slowly … but that never happened.

While taking care of her I learnt a lot about myself and how far I had come in my journey with mental illness.

When the department took my own babies away all those years ago, I had had to learn how to live without them every day. It forced me to take notice of what was going on for me and pay attention to my triggers.

It was an excruciating and painful time in life and a lot of the same feelings of not being good enough are under the surface, but I'm just better at hiding it now than I was before. When I look back at this time in life I am grateful that I was strong enough to come through it all and turn my life around.

At the same time as the foster baby left us I got the amazing and very surprising news that my 11 year old son had nominated me as The Barnardos Mother Of The Year and that I was the winner for Victoria!

He hadn't told me that he had entered the nomination and the news came as a shock to both of us. The media attention was INSANE! When you have low self-esteem and don't like attention at all, this was quite hard to keep standing in the light and smile. It was everywhere I turned.

The newspapers, on the radio, on the television and even on social media.

It was part of the celebrations I know, but the comments from those closest to me are what hurt the most.

My mother, my sister, my brothers ... they all had something to say. They refused to see that I had changed, that people can turn their lives around and make a difference to people's lives.

They tore me down on social media and then their friends started joining in. My son saw the comments and tried to hide the hurt from me, but it wasn't long before we both couldn't hold back the tears anymore.

We had to go up to Sydney for the national event that would name the overall winner of Mother Of The Year, and although we had never been before, the excitement was overshadowed by the hate and bullying that was going on behind the scenes.

I think I knew that this was finally it; that I had to once and for all stand up for myself and my boys and cut my mother and siblings out of my life completely.

No matter what they hurled at me via text message or private message, I replied simply with 'I hope that the rest of life treats you well.

Maybe one day you will see what you have done and see the hurt that it has caused. You won't hear from us again.'

It took me 4 hours to write those words and another 2 hours to hit send. For me it was the last thing I was ever going to communicate with them and I didn't want it to be words that were said in anger, hurt or pain. It was just an ending to 38 years of heartache that had never been apologized for.

Learning to live without a goodbye or sorry is hard sometimes and the thought has crossed my mind a few times to just pick up the phone and call them; but I can't this time.

In the back of my mind I have the same thing repeating over and over 'why can't my mother be proud of me?' 'what did I do to her that has made her think that I am not worthy of the love a child deserves from a parent?'.

A few years ago this would have sent me into a down ward spiral that only a stint in hospital would have fixed.

Not letting the negativity win proves to me how far I have come in the last 10 years.

I've talked friends out of suicide and stayed up for hours when they felt like the rest of the world had forgotten that they were there. I've given my boys a loving home and hugs for no reason so that they know what love feels like. I've fallen down many times but gotten up every time, and while I was doing it I showed them that life is always going to hit you with curve balls but that doesn't mean you have to stay down.

The proudest moment in my life to date was in February this year; the day that I got my final accreditation as a foster carer. There was no way I could hold back the tears! It took me almost two years of fighting a system that was much like my family, intent on having my history and past mistakes thrown back in my face. But in the end I got the answers I was looking for and along the way changed the policy and legislation around the criteria for future foster carers in Victoria.

Previously, if you had involvement from the department with your children and they were removed from your care, regardless of the reasons, you were automatically rejected to proceed with our application to foster.

When they asked me for character references and letters of support I got them. They asked for mental health assessments and I passed each and every one. When they asked me for my life story I gave it to them and held nothing back. Even when the memories surfaced of me being abused as a child, I was able to rise above it and talk about it without falling into a heap.

When they ran out of things to ask for I got the yes that I had worked so hard for.

CHRONIC PAIN – MY LIFE TODAY

For as long as I can remember I have always had chronic pain. As a teenager I was diagnosed with an hereditary condition called Schumann's disease, it caused my spine to become brittle and any exertion would leave me bedridden or in extreme pain. It wasn't easy to explain, and everyone just assumed I was making it up and bullied me for being overweight.

School was never fun! At 14 I was diagnosed with PCOS, poly cystic ovarian syndrome after needing emergency surgery for a burst cyst that had sent my stomach septic. I almost died on the table from the infection and regularly needed laparoscopic surgery to remove the cysts and help ease the pain of scar adhesions.

My weight has always been an issue for me and no matter what I did nothing worked. Bullying was something I learned to live with but that didn't mean it never hurt. Every year my birthday wish when I blew out the candles was to be skinny and popular like Amanda Thompson, a girl I went to school with and was everyone's dream girl.

It didn't help that my mother always pointed out that I was bigger than all the other girls when we were shopping for clothes or at Christmas time when my brothers and sisters woke up to sacks full or overflowing of stuff from santa and my sack would be a quarter full of clothes. Her reply was always the same, your clothes cost more because you are big. I learnt pretty quick to stop asking for things and to stop asking questions.

When I got pregnant at 17 it wasn't just a surprise, it was a miracle. I had heard so many doctors tell my parents that because I had PCOS my fertility had been affected.

So despite what everyone said. I decided to keep my baby. Even when my mother drove me to the family planning clinic and shoved $200 in my hand and told me to get out of the car and not come home till I had 'taken care of it'.

She told the baby's father that it wasn't his and had everyone believe that I had been sleeping around. His reaction was to threaten to take the baby and run, he had money and I didn't so I felt like I had nowhere to turn and decided to not name him on the birth certificate.

My son used to ask who his father was and I always told him that when he turned 18 I would tell him, but at 18 he told me he didn't want to know. Told me that now that he can know, he doesn't want to. I respect that and unless he asks again I will take that knowledge to my grave with me. Some people might judge me for that decision, but this is how it is and the rest of this story is not mine to tell.

Obviously I didn't 'get rid of it' as my mother had demanded and I've never told my son about that part of my story, and as much as I have wanted to since he went to live with her, I couldn't hurt him like that. But I have no doubt that had it been something for her to tell him she would have, in the hope that it would drive a wedge between me and my son.

She's an extremely toxic and volatile woman my mother. I often ask myself why I got her as a parent.

After I had my second son I was diagnosed with endometriosis and this is when my chronic pain kicked into high gear. Every day was a struggle, and little by little my quality of life was taken over with managing the pain.

All the doctors I saw seemed to think that if I lost weight then the pain would disappear! Like, the size of my uterus was going to change because I lost weight?! Seriously?!

For years I struggled with pain and got to a point where I was needing 30 tablets a day just to manage and be a mother to my boys. The pain was never gone, it was always there and some days were worse than others but unless I was screaming in agony I would do my best at home and not go to the hospital.

After our return from Sydney my pain escalated to a 10/10 and I went into hospital 4 times in a month to get relief from it.

I was treated like shit and told I was an addict just there seeking hard drugs. My symptoms to them were me 'detoxing' and not pain related. Withering on the floor in the fetal position, screaming and begging for them to end it wasn't enough, so they sent me home. Twice.

I went to the local paper with my story and although again the bullies came out in force and supported the hospitals decision to refuse me treatment, I got the operation I needed.

I had a total hysterectomy on September 1st and since the recovery I have a quality of life now that was nonexistent before. I don't need medication and I have lost 30 kilos.

I've changed my diet to vegan and cut out all sugar. No soft drink, meat, dairy or eggs and the changes in all of us (the kids are vegan by choice too!) is pretty insane! The odd bully is out there still but at least now I can smile when they say stuff because I am in control this time round.

WHAT DOES DEPRESSION LOOK LIKE?

Is depression the tears, frown, red puffy eyes from crying for so long?

Or the dark sketchy images of sitting in a corner or alone in a room covered in memories?

Take a look at the pictures below. Yep!...that's me.

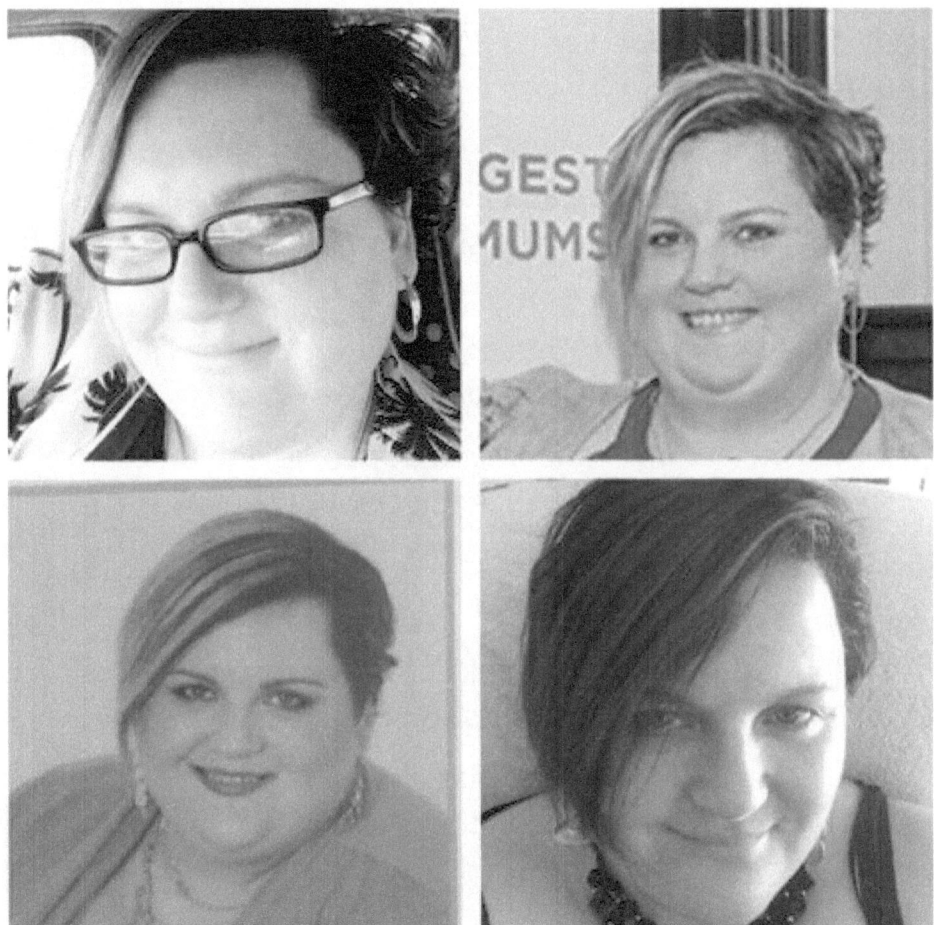

Would it surprise you to know that all 4 of these faces are depression and what it's like for me?

In the first photo I'm suffering from severe paranoia.

In the second photo I have depression.

In the bottom left side photo I have anxiety.

In the bottom right photo I have BPD.

They all represent one thing ... mental illness.

What You Do Not See Is What Depression Is Really About

It's smiling in spite of the tears that are brimming on the surface. It's the smiling at a public event and thinking to myself "please hurry and finish because I need a moment alone to cry"?

It's a smiling face with glasses on so that the suns glare doesn't capture the tears that are there?

It's the changed hair colour so that people don't look in to your eyes, and only notice the colour change? It's all of them.

This is me with mental illness.

You don't see the panic attacks or the tears that come from nowhere and take hours sometimes to leave.

You don't see the thoughts that are in my head, sometimes screaming so loud that even a whisper can sound so loud.

You can't see my hands that are shaking or my uneasy steps as I walk away from a situation that terrifies me.

You don't see how I scream into my pillow at night so that my children don't hear me cry, or the tears I cry in the shower when I'm rocking back and forth on the floor.

You don't hear my lies when you ask me if I'm okay and I answer 'I'm fine'.

You don't see the bruises I have or the cuts that I hide from the times when depression almost won.

The risks that I take, sometimes daily, just to feel SOMETHING instead of the pain.

You just don't 'see' depression. It's not that simple.

I have thoughts of suicide every single day and I have panic attacks that leave me exhausted for hours.

I still catch up with friends and I still laugh and support them when they need it too. I can go to work (most of the time) and look after my kids and myself, but that doesn't mean I'm better because I still have mental illness.

I can talk others out of suicide because I know exactly how they feel and I can be strong when my children need me to be, but sometimes I can't be strong for myself.

THIS is what depression "looks" like.

PLEASE don't judge people for what you can't see.

MISTY DARKNESS

In times of darkness the misty fog envelopes me.
There is stillness in the air.
There is quiet in the emptiness.
Alone in a world where everything is hidden in the mist;
It almost feels like I'm the only one left.
But then I hear them.
Quietly at first they talk,
Then it's a screaming war inside my mind!
The bare branches of the tree are a reflection of how stripped I feel of my identity.
The judgements, the attacks, the brutality of public opinion.
Solitude is begging me.
Sanity is leaving.
How does it all go so horribly wrong?
When will all start to again make sense?
Frozen inside from rejections of life.
Barely finding the energy to breathe.
Self-inflicted and guilty as sin,
Nothing is happening.
Don't think I can win ...

UNWANTED VISITOR

I started up a small business about 9 months ago. Every waking hour I poured myself into creating new pieces for my collection. Used to wake up and be inspired at what would come from the day's activities.

The last few weeks the Crafts have been left gathering dust on the table, my jars are sitting in the cupboard, forgotten, untouched and some are even broken. I've been going for days without having a shower, making promises that I'll do it tomorrow. Serving up shitty food as the nightly meal to my kids and I think I made my bed last week, or maybe it was the week before ...

I stopped styling my hair a while ago. Just too hard to straighten it every day, so I just wrap it in scarves and hope for the best or use a headband to hold it back.

There is so much washing in the laundry room that we have to throw it in and hope for the best! Hope the door closes behind us. I'm almost positive someone spilled milk somewhere ... it's slowly stinking up the place. When I wake up these days I count slowly to ten.

1 - I'm alive
2 - are the kids awake yet
3 - what part of me hurts the most
4 - do I have time to have a nap
5 - how long can I lay here for
6 - I'm definitely still alive
7 - am I happy about that fact?
8 - if I get up & pee will it wake them up?
9 - is it still dark out?
10 - do I really need to get out of bed yet?

Most days I end up crying because one of the thousand things bothering me just gets too much, and I've stopped trying to turn them off.

When people see me they wouldn't have a clue and don't see what's really inside. I laugh, I smile, sometimes I even get things done, but the effort it takes to even step outside is exhausting to say the least!

Sometime during the last few weeks someone came to stay with us. Turned up uninvited and decided to just move in. I've tried to get them to leave! Bribed, bargained, begged and pleaded with them to go, but even that has become too hard so we just kind of co-exist together. I hate that they're back after a long time away and I'm not afraid to admit but I'm kinda scared to have them here. I never said it was a friend never agreed to have it here, but now that it is I've got to send it away somehow. But I can't remember how I can do that when it's taken so much from me already.

My desire to keep on building my business, the joy from being a mum. The simple things that life was once full of. I just realised I forgot to introduce you! This thing that's moved right in and taken over. But don't worry one bit that they will come visit you too.

For me I say 'hello my old friend' but to you it's called depression.

SOMETIMES I FAIL

I failed at being a good mum today.

I raised my voice, I yelled and screamed. I cried and I fell apart at least a dozen times. I was mean and nasty and I don't even know why.

Master 5 pissed me off by defiantly saying NO to everything he was asked to do. Moody Mr 13 wouldn't come out of his room so I took away his laptop & his tv.

I tried to reason with everyone but lost my shit when they didn't wanna hear it.

I was gonna cook dinner but burnt the damn lasagna, so that was cancelled. We had toast instead. Master 5 has major attitude and pisses everyone off, then my old friends guilt and anxiety came to visit and wore out their welcome all by 10am!

Did I say things that I didn't mean? Yes.

Did I hurt my kids feelings? Yes.

Did I mean what I said? No.

Did I apologise to them for being a horrible mum today? Yes.

I'm tired now but I can't sleep. I wanna wake the boys up just so I can hug them and tell them I'm sorry again. I want to slap my self for letting it all get the better of me. But most of all I want to go back to this morning and start today again; but this time be a nicer and more understanding mum.

My throat feels like it has a huge lump in it that won't let me breathe and the tears I'm trying to hold back are sliding down my face despite how tightly I've shut my eyes.

Why was I so mean?

Why did I say such awful things?

When did I become my mother?!

I'm standing at the edge of the cliff with my boys faces staring at me full of hurt from things I've said today on one side and on the other a reflection of my mother staring back at me ... I want to just close my eyes and have it all go away, but all I can do is step back away from the edge and promise myself that tomorrow will be different.

Today I failed at being a good mum and it hurts me because I know that I'm better than this.

I yelled because I was frustrated.

I said nasty things because I was hurting.

I took things away because I was feeling ignored.

I was screaming because I was tired of talking.

And I was mean because I was exhausted.

I failed at being a good mum today.

HELP

The last month or so I've been dragged down by depression. It's begged me to follow down its painful path, and tempted me with thoughts that I'd rather not have to say. If not for a few very beautiful kind hearted souls, I would never have made it through.

I'm still fighting every single day to get back to my Old Self again, but it's just so hard when it feels like you are the only one fighting.

I'm having panic attacks every day and dread having to leave my house.

My anxiety gets the better of me most days, but slowly I'm finding my way back.

When I've needed some help, some support and some love, I've been lucky enough to have friends close by that think nothing of coming to be by my side. I sometimes forget how quickly it all takes over, how it throws you so fast that you're afraid it will break you when you finally fall.

I've thought about suicide at least once every day and I've distracted myself from the pain. Thank God for my friends that really are more like my family, it's been so very hard to keep the demons away. You will never realise how many times you've saved me, from myself and from the thoughts that so quickly can become reactions.

Never forget how much I love you. I'm blessed to call you my friends and always know that I'm here for you too. Together always until the end.

I know I'm gonna be fine, everything will be okay again one day because I know these demons that have woken up inside me weren't expecting the army that I have waiting.

BI POLAR

It's been a long time since I've felt like this. Lost, sad, angry and afraid to go out anywhere.

My moods have been erratic and I've not wanted to talk to anyone.

I went and saw my GP and he's put me on medication.

Just when I finally come to terms with my BPD diagnosis ... I then get another 'label' and this time it's Bipolar.

All that keeps going through my head is 'oh for fuck sakes! What next?!' I'm still not convinced - but that may just be my way of putting off the inevitable!

For now all I can do is take it one day at a time and hope that things will start getting easier in the future.

Walk with me awhile so I'm not doing this alone?

Thank you ❤️❤️ I love you ❤️

I'm smiling in the photos people take. I'm laughing at the funny things people say to me. I'm doing everything that I need to do, but I feel so empty inside.

It's more than loneliness; it's more than wanting to have someone beside me to talk to, and it's more than just going through the motions of getting up and getting through the day.

Can you miss something you never had?

Sometimes I find myself watching the clock as if I'm waiting for something to happen, like suddenly it's 'THAT TIME' and everything changes and my life is full again.

Some days I feel brilliant. I can get out and do things and not give a single fuck about what others think when they look at me; other days I have zero energy. I can barely get out of bed. Have no energy to speak or move, can't even be referee when the kids are ready to kill each other. I try and force myself to do things.

Sometimes anything just so that I'm busy, but the effort of forcing it all makes it harder to do anything.

It feels like I woke up one day and just felt like something inside me was gone and in its place is emptiness.

I have no idea what it was or is, no clue how or where to find it to replace it and every day it ever so slightly just grows a little more.

I'm empty inside and it's swallowing me whole. The lump in my throat is choking me most days and my anger is growing into a forest fire. But it's the 'nothing' that bothers me most.

JUST BREATHE...

It feels like I'm suffocating on air.
The dense humidity sucks the breath from my lungs
And I'm choking on what's left behind.
Hands around my neck only grasp harder the more I try and fight it.
Reaching out for something to hold,
Scared that I'm going under
And knowing if I do this time;
There is no coming back.
Treading water and getting nowhere near the shore;
My head screams at me to stop
But giving up is not an option!
Holding it all in as waves pound down on top of me,
And humidity sucking it out of my every breath.
Choking and gagging all at once
And my legs are giving in.
Frozen in fear.
Frozen in fight.
Still beneath me; even though I'm telling them to not give up.
Time stands still and it's time to decide.
Do I go under?
Or keep trying to hold on?
It feels like my feet are encased in cement, no longer feeling;
Not even numb.

My lungs are full of stolen air and the humidity is still choking me.

I'm too tired now to even care.

So I'm just gonna close my eyes and hope that when I open them,

Somehow; I'll know what I have to do.

DEPRESSION STARTED SLEEPING

Depression started sleeping.
Depression started emotional eating.
Depression started nightmares.
Depression started crying.
Depression started up the little voice again.
Depression started self hatred and doubt.
Depression started to wipe me out.
Depression started messing with me head.
Depression I know it wants me ....
Dead.
Dead.
Dead.

LAST WEEK....

Last week this was me. I couldn't shake the darkness that was covering me. Every single thing in my life was weighing down my motivation, my mind, body and soul.

Nights were long and lonely and the darkness was everywhere I turned. I couldn't speak or tell anyone just how bad it really was because I knew that I was going to get 'the look', so I stayed silent.

The days were long but filled with sadness and regret that I couldn't find the energy to move and do a single thing even when I knew the list was long.

I was so so tired, but felt like I couldn't sleep; but then just as quickly as sleep had eluded me, it took all I had just to keep my eyes open. Nothing made me happy, nothing made me want to stop falling into the hole that I'd fallen into. Nothing was making me want to stay even when I had so much I had to live for.

Today; I'm awake and very happy to be me and to look at me you'd never know that only days ago I was a mess on the bathroom floor with the music turned up loud so that the kids couldn't hear me cry, You'd not see the darkness that was following me everywhere, suffocating me for having life.

It doesn't take much for it to weave its way back in. Every day I fight it off. Sometimes I am stronger and can have a better today, tomorrow or next week. Other times nothing that I do will work and I find that it's gotten in.

It's not cured, it's not gone, it's not anywhere but it's everywhere. It's just a part of me that makes me, me.

In 2007 I attempted suicide by sitting in my car in a closed garage with a hose in the tailpipe.

I had no idea if I was doing it right but I had seen it in a movie once, so thought that was easy and painless and how I chose to leave this life.

I don't remember much of what happened but I did answer a phone call and vaguely remember hearing sirens in the distance as I lost consciousness.

At the time, I didn't care that I might have problems with my memory and fought the doctors at every turn. I pulled my oxygen mask off and wouldn't do the breathing exercises they were giving me. Everything they told me I laughed at. Didn't realise how close to had come to causing myself major irreversible damage and death and quite frankly I didn't care.

How I regret my decision now.

I've never told anyone about this next part. Not a soul.

11 years later and have big pieces of my past missing. Some things I can remember in intricate detail, then other things I have no memory of at all. When people talk about people from my past, a lot of times I remember them as they were years ago and seeing photos of them older and grown my brain struggles to connect the image with how I last saw them.

Some days; especially when I'm tired or stressed I stumble over simple words or can't remember names for things like salt and pepper.

When it first started happening a few years ago I put it down the meds I was on for my anxiety, but I eventually took my doctors' advice and has some tests done.

I have some long term and short term memory loss that gets worse when I'm tired. Can't undo what's been done so I try to write things down as I remember them.

I regret fighting the doctors and wish that there was a way to turn back the clock to the moment I turned the ignition that day in a locked garage; but we both know that that can't happen.

I guess if I've learned anything from this it's that your memories are what keep you company. Constantly a constant. When you lose them, you lose a small part of who you are, so try to keep them safe.

SOMETIMES I MISS MY SUICIDE

Sometimes I miss my suicide,
When I was in control.
It wasn't hard, it didn't hurt
I just remember being afraid.
A bit like now my demons wake
And strip my reality
So it all feels fake.

Sometimes I miss my suicide,
When I was in control.
It wasn't hard, it didn't hurt
I just remember being afraid.
I hear them laughing at all my faults
I hear them calling my name at night,
Telling me that they just know the way to make everything alright.

Sometimes I miss my suicide,
When I was in control.
It wasn't hard, it didn't hurt
I just remember being afraid.
I wake each day to new bruises,
How I got them is unclear,
I simply assume they are really real - And then they disappear.

Hannah Dee

Sometimes I miss my suicide,
When I was in control.
It wasn't hard, it didn't hurt
I just remember being afraid.
It happens all so sudden,
The darkness that surrounds me and holds me like a vice
Whispers softly 'what's the price?'

Sometimes I miss my suicide,
When I was in control.
It wasn't hard, it didn't hurt
I just remember being afraid.
The haunting by my enemy follows me everywhere,
It's not my friend, it's not my foe,
It's always there and will not go.

Sometimes I miss my suicide
When I was in control.
It wasn't hard, it didn't hurt.
I just remember being afraid.
Staying's not the question, I know I'm needed here.
But this demon monster wears me down;
Till I jump at my own shadow and my hands just shake in fear.

Sometimes I miss my suicide,
When I was in control.
It wasn't hard, it didn't hurt,
I just remember feeling afraid.
Again it whispers 'what's your price' and I'm crying from the fear.
But I stand up tall and fill my lungs and scream
'you're not welcome here'!

Sometimes I miss my suicide
When I was in control.
It wasn't hard, it didn't hurt,
I just remember being afraid.
My mind is down to a quite lull And I think I've won this war.
But I've no doubt, of this I'm sure
The monsters, and demons keep the score.

Every day I think about suicide.

It's always niggling at the back of my mind. Sometimes I even entertain the ideas I have about how I would do it.

But, although I think about suicide, it doesn't mean I want to die.

Part of my illness means that I have suicidal ideation.

Many years ago I would struggle with the constant thoughts I was having and thought the only way to silence them was to do them. But when it came down to it, in the lead up to it, I'd realise that it wasn't what I wanted after all.

Eventually, after years of educating myself and learning how to function with these thoughts in my mind I have found a safe place. I can have the thoughts, I can sit with them and not act on them and still be able to go about my day without them getting too much time and attention.

They don't control me anymore like they once did.

I still have times when they get really loud and drag me down, begging me to listen. But calling on my supports helps get me back on track.

DEMONS

Wasn't one of hers that was chasing her down, but the sound of her unsteady breath and the screams she was trying to stifle that made him run faster. He was feeding on her terror like it was his own. Finally when he caught up he smiled. A twisted, crooked smile of delight. For this time he was sure he had her!

But when he touched her arm while turning her from the light, he gasped and dropped his hand back at his side.

It was only then that she realized her demons, the ones that lived inside of her .. had caused her enough pain already. And that this demon, who had chased her down, intending to be a torturer to her soul ...knew only too well, simply by touching her for only a slight second .. that she has already fought enough battles and wasn't strong enough to fight anymore.

He hadn't wanted a victim, just someone to mess around with. To beg him to stop. He'd only wanted a bit of fun.

As far as demons go, with inflicting pain upon the tortured, he was really just a pussy cat and never did any lasting damage.

So he left her there on the spot where the dark met with the light. But when he turned to look back over his shoulder ... She was gone.

And he heard her demons laughing with delight.
They had won.

FOSTER CARE

At 10.17am April 11th she left.

The overwhelming sadness that enveloped me as the car pulled away from the curb hit me like a tonne of bricks.

I lost the ability to stand and I fell to the ground, my screams too painful to keep inside. My heart broke in two, I swear I felt the exact moment that it happened and I started to cry. Big heavy tears soaked my sleeves and I didn't care who saw me there on the side of the road rocking back and forth. I couldn't breathe, my lungs were so tight and my anguished cries turned into painful howls.

I stayed like this for almost an hour before I could pick myself up again.

Now it feels like my emotions have turned off. I feel numb and like I'm in a dream, walking up to her room and packing up more of her toys.

Auto pilot has kicked in because reality is just too much to bear. I keep expecting to hear her little giggle as she comes up the hallway to find me, hear the slap, slap of her little hands hitting the carpet. But then I remember that she's not here anymore.

My head has started pounding and my eyes are so red and puffy; surely they will never go back to normal again?

This is cruel. So, so cruel. It's not completely sunk in yet that this is real.

She's gone.

She's gone.

Suddenly my arms are empty, the room is empty, the house feels so big and empty without her in it. I don't know if I will ever get over it. I didn't sign up for this and I didn't expect that I'd fall so hard, but did I have another choice? Should I never have let her stay?

I don't know how I'm meant to go on now and fill my days. Can't remember what I did before she came into my life.

For 47 weeks and 4 days I proved to everyone, including myself that I could do it.

And I did a damn good job raising her!

Fuck the system.

This time they got it wrong.

And I honestly don't think that I can do this again ....

You were my first foster baby. Eleven months of undeniable happiness you brought into my world.

You were my first awakening to the love that I never knew I had in me to share with anyone other than my own babies.

Oh how I will remember you.

The way your eyes would light up when you saw me in the mornings, always made my heart sing.

Your little fingers wrapped around my own as you fell asleep in my now empty arms. I will never forget how that made me feel.

The moments when you were insecure and distressed and searched my eyes for a sign that it was all going to be okay

I will never forget it - ever.

The way my belly churned in knots at the thought of you leaving, so I held you a little tighter; For just awhile longer.

You might not remember me. You Might grow up and never remember my name.

But I hope that you know that you were loved so very dearly. And always will be by me.

From the moment you came into my life, I knew that you were special.

No matter where you go, what you do, what life throws your way, always, always remember that there is someone out there that loves you and thinks of you every day.

Our journey may have come to an end my darling girl, but never doubt that with your leaving my heart will never be the same.

Because in the deepest part, that's now locked away there is a hole that only you can fill.

Your footprint is imprinted there. Now and Forever you will always be part of me along with the memories we have made.

Be brave. Be strong. Be amazing Missy moo

But most of all ... Just Be You.

For Little Missy Moo

They didn't tell me not to love you.
Look after her, they said.
Care for her; they said.
Tell her that you'll protect her.
Hold her. Feed her.
Show her that you care.
Soothe her when she cries.
Change her when she's dirty.
Tell her that you care.

They asked me if I'd take you in and keep you safe from harm.
Do everything a mother does, but don't you dare be a mother to her!
I kept you safe. I took you in.
I gave you a home.
I showed you what a family looks like.
I dried your tears. I calmed your fears.
I treated you as my own.
But no one ever told me. Not a single living soul.
They didn't tell me not to love you.
But I have, I did, I always will.

Now that you are leaving.
It's so hard to let you go.
My heart is feeling broken.
And I know it always will.
They didn't tell me not to love you.
They didn't tell me not to love.
They didn't tell me not to.

They didn't tell me not.
They didn't tell me.
They didn't tell.
They didn't.

Loving you like you are one of my own is easy to do when your hearts been hurt a few too many times before.

The 3am feeds when the world is dark and sleeping are some of my favourite moments. It's like no one else exists, no one else matters because I've got you and you've got me. I don't want another human being on earth to feel the way I have done before. The sadness and the hurt, the pain that life has throws you way sometimes ... It will either make you or it will break you so they say.

My eyes are getting heavy, yours are too, but we still have time for a smile or two before you drift back off to sleep in my arms again.

I get to love you. The magnitude and sadness of that single word 'love' is not lost on my heart. I get to learn from you about just how strong my heart can be, because one day I'll have to let you go and if it's not strong enough, then it's gonna break.

Every time a new little one comes in through the door I fall in love with them too, just as I did with you. And before they leave ... they fall in love just a little, even a tiny bit with me too.

That's always just enough to fill me up with all the love I need to pick myself back up and love again tomorrow.

Now the time reads 4am and you've been sleeping for the past hour, but I want to hold you a moment longer so I've not got any regrets.

Because every time when the little ones leave, I ask myself a single question. 'Why didn't I hold them for just another moment more?'

So I take them when I can get them, kiss you ever so lightly as I put you back into bed, then whisper goodnight and tell you that I'm gonna see you again soon.

With my heart now full again I climb into bed and fall asleep ready to do it all again in just a few short hours.

Because when you find your purpose in life; you've found you.

Behind The Mask

It's closing your eyes for just a moment,

It's washing out bottles & cleaning dishes at 3am,

It's changing nappies,

It's putting on yet another load of washing.

It's drying tears,

It's holding them tight,

It's loving them,

It's being there for them,

It's being so tired you can't think straight,

It's getting back up when you just sat down,

It's not knowing if it's gonna work, it's taking the risk that it will anyway.

It's juggling school lunches,

It's driving in peak hour traffic,

It's needing to be in 3 places at once,

It's being referee,

It's being a cheerleader,

It's about doing your best,

It's about being the someone they need.

It's about taking a moment to take it all in,

It's about helping them,

It's about giving them a part of yourself,

It's about sometimes getting very little in return,

It's about the effort that makes it count.

It's life,

It's unexpected,

It's challenging,

It's rewarding,

It's sometimes thankless,

It's definitely hard,

It's sadness,

It's happiness,

It's chaos,

It's calm.

It's them,

It's knowing that what you do counts.

It's listening,

It's caring,

It's everything and much much more.

It's being braver than thought that you'd ever need to be.

It's being tired & wanting to give up,

It's hanging in there a moment more.

It's making the moments count,

It's about stepping up when their world has fallen apart.

This is me.

LABELS

Some say that I couldn't possibly love someone else's child as much as I love my own. Some say that I'm not cut out for it. Some say that it's going to hurt, so that fear stops them from ever trying. Some say that I'm not her mother so I should keep her at arm's length so that she doesn't get confused.

I say, loving her is the easy part. She may not be biologically mine, but she's my daughter. Why should she be treated as anything else? She's 10 months old. Lived with me more than half of her life. When she is sick, I hold her and kiss her till she's better. I take her to the doctor and hold her tight when she's feeling unsure and afraid. I buy her clothes, cook her food. Syringe feed her when she's too weak to drink. Get up countless times at night to settle her when she's teething. I play with her, I teach her things. I cry with her and am afraid for her. I lay awake at night wondering if this next court date will be the one that changes everything.

I send pictures and updates to her parents and I ask their permission when I need to take her places. When she first came to live with us at 10 weeks old, I used to correct people and say 'she's a foster baby' when they said 'oohhh she looks like her brother' but then I would see the pity in people's eyes and I thought that's not fair on her. She doesn't need pity from people. She needs love, and acceptance for who she is, exactly as she is. It shouldn't take the word 'foster' to evoke those feelings from people, so I've stopped saying it.

She has shown me a great strength that I didn't know I had. By loving and caring ... no ... raising her I have learnt how to be more compassionate, to be more empathetic towards others and to be a better parent to my children. Treating them all as equals shows them that they are still loved. No better, no worse than her. They play together, they argue, they look out for each other, But most importantly they all love each other.

Raising children in a loving and safe environment shouldn't be dictated by the words 'foster care' because all children DESERVE to have both those things regardless. So yes - biologically I'm not her mother, and nothing will ever change that. But while she's here living with us and growing, learning, and exploring what life is all about ... I'm her Mum. Her security. Her stability. Her everything in her world that makes it right. If that still leaves you debating that I'm her Mum in any way, then I guess we have to agree to disagree. Because DNA has got nothing to do with it.

HOW LABELS MAKE YOU FEEL

How many of you feel that you are not entitled to the same as everyone else because of your illness? How many times have you seen an opportunity but not tried to cease the moment because of your illness? Is it holding you back? Is it making you doubt what you can do?

It did me. Every single day I doubted myself and kept telling myself that I couldn't, shouldn't or wouldn't do something because there was this thing that was wrong with me. I let my labels become me. I wasn't Hannah the Mum, I was a Mum with mental health issues. The lady who can't work because of her mental health. That lady with the issues. My labels were all that anyone knew me as and that was because I had let them take over who I was.

It's not easy to do, but I found a way to use it to my advantage. The hospital that I had been in the psych ward at was looking for users of the device to give feedback on how to improve it. Given that I had a complexity of issues, problems & opinions I decided that the only way that they will know about all this stuff is if I tell them. So I did and it felt good to finally use my experiences to help make things better for someone else. I was later asked to join a committee with other people with mental health conditions. This was where I found my voice again and was able to give my experiences a purpose. I am now currently sitting on 4 different committees within the Victorian mental health sector and also do public speaking at forums and events that highlight the strengths that we all have.

I've been a state winner for Mother of the year and now an accredited foster carer for children 5 and under, never did I ever think in my times of darkness and complete and utter dispair that this would be my life today. In fact had someone even suggested it I would have laughed and told them to quit dreaming!!

People that work in mental health now know my name and ask me to consult with them on new legislation, I still pinch myself sometimes because it all feels like a dream!

My labels are still the same. I have diagnosed BPD, depression, anxiety & Bi-polar. Difference now though is that I am Hannah first, my labels are just part of who I am. If I can survive 22 suicide attempts and a successful suicide that had me clinically dead for 3 minutes … then I am meant to be here right?

Who I am today is my purpose in life. From now until I no longer have the ability to do it, I will keep doing what I do and love to help others get access to a fairer system.

Your voice matters.

Your life experience is priceless.

Your labels make up part of who you are.

I believe in you.

FRIENDS

The last month or so I've been dragged down by depression. It's begged me to follow down its painful path, and tempted me with thoughts that I'd rather not have to say. If not for a few very beautiful kind hearted souls, I would never have made it through.

I'm still fighting every single day to get back to my Old self again, but it's just so hard when it feels like you are the only one fighting. I'm having panic attacks every day and dread having to leave my house. My anxiety gets the better of me most days, but slowly I'm finding my way back. When I've needed some help, some support and some love, I've been lucky enough to have friends close by that think nothing of coming to be by my side.

I sometimes forget how quickly it all takes over; how it throws you so fast that you're afraid it will break you when you finally fall. I've thought about suicide at least once every day and I've distracted myself from the pain. Thank god for my friends that really are more like my family, it's been so very hard to keep the demons away.

You will never realise how many times you've saved me, from myself and from the thoughts that so quickly can become reactions. Never forget how much I love you. I'm blessed to call you my friends and always know that I'm here for you too. Together always until the end. I know I'm gonna be fine, everything will be okay again one day because I know these demons that have woken up inside me weren't expecting the army that I have waiting.

BEL

When I was in high school I didn't have many friends. I never had the right clothes for school, so I got picked on a lot.

I did have one friend though who was always there for me when the bullies got too loud or wouldn't stop their hatred towards me. Her name was Belinda and I was so happy when she walked up to the bullies one day and told them that I was her friend and if they had a problem with me then they had a problem with her.

From then on she always looked out for me and made sure that I was okay. We stayed in touch when we left school and I even helped her get a job at the store where I was working.

We used to hang out at each other's place and our babies were only a year apart but in 1998 my world came crashing down when I got the news she had been killed in a car accident.

I didn't know about this until an hour after it happened and in that time I had gotten upset with her for yet again letting me down and not showing up to dinner like she planned. I had left her a voice message saying 'This is the last time I invite you to dinner Bin! There's no excuse unless you are dead or dying for you to not call me and tell me you're not coming!'

Those words have haunted me for a very long time. I later found out what had happened and the pain of my words, although she never heard them, played over and over in my mind.

She was coming to my place for dinner, but she had a fight with her boyfriend before leaving and he had chased her and some friends she was dropping off down the street down a highway at high speed. As she had unbuckled her seatbelt to make a quick exit from the car as it stopped, his car smashed into hers and she was thrown out the front window.

She died on impact. I still miss her every day.

After her funeral the father of her son took him interstate and I never got to see him again. It was like a cruel game was played because it felt like I had lost both of them. She would have been 40 this year had she still been alive, but she is in my heart and will always be special to me for everything she did. She made life better, happier and funnier at a time when I needed it the most.

Today we should be celebrating your birthday.

There isn't a day that goes by when I don't miss you.

I tell you goodnight when I get into bed and I blow you a kiss when I'm leaving my room. You were my best friend.

There are so many things I want to tell you Bel, and so much gossip I just know we'd be giggling for hours!

Happy 39th Birthday my beautiful friend. I'm sure you're having a huge party up there and causing chaos as only you know how to do!

Your leaving so suddenly all those years ago taught me to never take anything for granted.

Love you always and forever darling girl 💗🖤💙🖤

A LIGHT AT THE END OF THE TUNNEL

The world can be dark and relentless with its pain, but you have been through so much now that this just feels like a dress rehearsal.

Sometimes it feels like the play has already started but your still stuck in wardrobe!

So walk out now .. And own it!

Without you it's just a pantomime.

Standing is the easy part.

It's the getting back up that's hard!

Making the decision to help someone you will never meet says a lot about your character.

Even if you can't see it today - the light is still shining ... So Instead of looking down, try looking up.

www.ingramcontent.com/pod-product-compliance
Lightning Source LLC
Chambersburg PA
CBHW020455220526
45464CB00002B/993